HIRING HIGH QUALITY EMERGENCY MEDICINE PHYSICIAN ASSISTANTS AND NURSE PRACTITIONERS:

HIRING HIGH QUALITY EMERGENCY MEDICINE PHYSICIAN ASSISTANTS AND NURSE PRACTITIONERS:

Finding the Right People and Retaining Talent

Gary Josephsen, MD

To my wife, thanks for giving me the job.

Contents

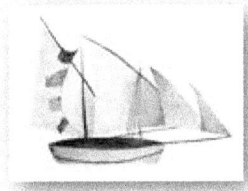

The Right and the Wrong Way to Hire

Once when I joined a group, the director sat me down for an orientation. "The profit structure is stepwise; we vote on partnership after the second year," he told me. "And you can't sleep with any of the registration clerks." I was caught off guard, but agreed not to sleep with any of them. This, it turns out, was the major problem with the physician I was hired to replace.

The physician who had been let go had done his residency with the current assistant director. They were friends. When they hired him, he had a reputation as a good clinician and good references, and he interviewed well. About a year into his time with the group, coworkers noticed that he was often gone for long periods of time while on shift. He would return to the department and resume his work without explanation. Eventually, one of the registration clerks became pregnant and quit soon thereafter. Another female clerk was seen necking with him in the parking lot. The hospital administration started getting complaints from other staff members that one of the ED doctors was using the ED doctors' office to have sex while on duty. It was a problem.

He left without incident, but at about the same time, another doctor seemed to be having a lot of cases go through quality review. Fresh out of residency, it was assumed that he needed some guidance and a little extra time with the books, so the group gave him some feedback. He seemed to take it well, and for a few months, his work improved. Then another string of cases cropped up, and the pattern repeated itself. But because he was such a nice guy and so loved by the nursing staff, no one, myself included, wanted to let him go. The group formed a professional review committee to meet and try to mentor him, but the quality of his care just never seemed to get better for very long. His progress just wasn't consistent. Finally, the group leveled with him: his care was dangerous, and he could no longer practice with the group. He left and filed a lawsuit against the group. The combined investment in hiring, mentoring, reviewing, and firing him was enormous. Time dedicated to the legal battle continues to add up. It will go on for years.

It's easy to hire wrong. When ED staffing is short, the search begins for a new doctor or emergency medicine advanced practice provider (which will be abbreviated as EMAPP from here on, in the text), indicating a physician assistant or nurse practitioner. This book will primarily focus on EMAPPs because of the complexity associated with finding and training them, and the high level of turnover they see compared with physicians. But for any hire, regardless of position, there are consequences for doing it wrong.

Hiring mistakes are a massive waste of time. Usually, the assistant director of a group is responsible for staffing. This great responsibility generally comes to physicians with minimal training or experience in hiring. It takes time: time to search, advertise, interview, sell, evaluate, and train. Then, when it is time to terminate staff, it takes time to repeat the process all over again. And when someone doesn't work out, this person will also need to correspond with all the new groups looking to hire the person he or she just let go. This means more time wasted on the phone and in correspondence—time that can never be recovered.

The hiring process can also be a money pit. Advertising is becoming more expensive as those who run the internet job boards realize EM groups will spend more money to find the right person. Markups of 1,000 percent aren't uncommon for job advertisements. When new people join the group, they usually start slow, which hobbles productivity, leaving others to pick up the slack. The new hire's training eats up productivity that could be spent on patient care in the ED, practicing medicine. In addition to lost productivity, the cost from a single wrongful termination lawsuit can be devastating. And such costs aren't covered by malpractice insurance.

Hiring mistakes are also an emotional drain. Finding the right people can be difficult. As we will see, the traditional interview doesn't really provide the practical information necessary for choosing one applicant over another. Choosing the right person is stressful. When we choose an applicant and recruit the person to our group, we make an emotional investment. We spend time, money, and lots of effort to train and orient the new hire. Then, if it doesn't work out, we fire them. The loss aversion and emotional labor can blind us to their poor performance. No applicants want to relocate their family unless there is a high likelihood that they will succeed and be valued in their workplace. When it doesn't work out, anger and frustration can fuel hostility and legal action.

When the wrong person is hired, it also poses a professional risk to the group. We risk our reputation, contract loss for independent groups, and even the health of our patients. Hiring is something that we all need to do. And more of us need to do it right.

NONANALYTICAL HIRING: EVERYONE MAKES UP THEIR OWN RECIPE

Ask people how they hire, and you're likely to hear a lot of different answers. That's because there's tremendous variation and little training when it comes to hiring—especially in medicine.

Some people like to spend time asking applicants "tough questions." Like an interrogator, they want to see how the applicant will react under pressure. Others prefer avoiding confrontation in favor of casual conversation. If it goes well, they might assume the person will be easy to work with and that everything else can be learned on the job. Still other methods include bringing applicants to dinner to see how they get along with the other group members at a restaurant or bar. Sometimes, the group members themselves don't get along with each other during these interviews, even when they are on their best behavior. Other interviewers rely on trick questions to see what their interviewees are really like under their professional façade.

There are problems with each of these techniques, and yet they feel right, in part because our brains are wired for interpersonal interactions. We are social animals and generally pretty savvy ones. But the software of our brains, which evolved for life in small tribes, is poorly designed for complex decision making. And hiring is a complex decision.

HEURISTIC BIAS IN HIRING

As many readers know, the term *heuristic* refers to the shortcuts our brain takes when we make decisions quickly. Our brains have a tendency to take these shortcuts in three different ways.

One is that we tend to confirm our suspicions rather than come up with ways of disproving them. In the hiring process, we often allow ourselves to be led down the garden path in the interest of maintaining rapport with our applicant. Sometimes this is intentional. Other times, it is not.

We also tend to substitute one talent for another when judging competency. We suspect that the auto mechanic who talks slow might not be a good mechanic because we allow slow speech to imply slowness in other areas. In reality, his speech is not connected to his professional competency, and yet we allow our intuition to whisper lies in our ear. We gravitate toward articulate financial advisors, even though speeches don't help people invest. We sidle up in front of beautiful bartenders who can't pour drinks. In the ED, the recipe for success involves a specific set of skills that are not adequately evaluated in the typical interview process.

The third way our brains blind us during the interview process is through our tendency to over-rely on what is called *available information*. Daniel Kahneman, cognitive psychologist and Nobel laureate, calls this heuristic bias: "What you see is all there is," or WYSIATI, as he abbreviates it. When we have only some of the information we need, there is still a tendency toward overconfident decision making despite our limited information. For example, we meet an applicant who interviews well, and maybe we like them. We want to work with him or her. We also want to be fully staffed again. So when it's time to make reference calls, we underprepare, limit discussion, or sometimes (admit it) even skip some of the necessary reference calls altogether. And all of this is in spite of the fact that any one of those references might be able to tell us something that would lead us to cross the candidate off our list so fast the pencil would break.

A BETTER WAY TO HIRE

We can hire whomever we want. If you think an applicant will succeed, they may. You can take the risk if you're willing. But studies on hiring practices suggest that choosing candidates who are very likely to succeed limits turnover. So the question becomes, how do you find EMAPPs who have a 99 percent chance of success in your ED? And how do you avoid the consequences of a mis-hire? The extended training, repeated relocation, firing, malpractice, and other lawsuits are avoidable. You can avoid them by hiring skills, not people.

This dirty little secret of hiring is discouraging, but it's also liberating. Finding the right person for the job is a fool's errand. It's an impossible task. And when we do find what seems like a perfect fit, hindsight usually tells us there was a large amount of luck involved. This idea that it's nearly impossible to find the right people using standard job interview methods is unfashionable. But it's true.

Most strategies for hiring focus on finding the right person for the job. We like to believe that finding someone with the right disposition will solve our hiring problems, but social psychology suggests that an applicant's new job conditions are much more predictive of success than the disposition they bring to their job. For example, a highly qualified applicant might experience adverse work conditions that stand in the way of success. Or a mediocre candidate might forge a close connection with solid mentors who help the person learn the skills he or she needs. When it comes to success on the job, the work environment might be even more important than the person we put in the position.

But there's one problem with this thinking: no one really believes it. And the reason we don't believe it is because we are wired not to. This tendency has a name. When we tend to attribute a person's performance to their disposition rather than the situation, we commit the fundamental attribution error, a heuristic bias. This is not to say that a person's disposition has no effect on his or her chance of success; it's true that hardworking people tend to succeed. In the second chapter, we will see why predicting performance based on personality traits is nearly impossible.

So why should we put forth so much effort? Because it's usually the wrong people who are easily found. The perfect person for the position is difficult to assess in advance, but we can make things easier by eliminating some of the wrong people: Those who can't get along with others and those who habitually lie or take shortcuts, for instance. These people are easily screened out during the hiring process. It may be hard, however, to find people with the disposition to succeed because disposition may not be the key to their success. The environment you create for your new hires may allow for many types of people to succeed or fail, depending on your training and orientation process. What remains in the hiring process is to find applicants who are unlikely to work out. These people are not hard to identify, but weeding them out does involve some amount of hard work.

After you've identified all the wrong people, what remains is a relatively large group of applicants that could succeed in your position, given the right coaching. How easy will the process be on you and on them? That depends on the level of skill they bring to the job, how well their skills are suited to the position, and how much ground they will need to make up while acclimating to a new work environment.

Fortunately, emergency medicine demands a pretty well-defined skill set. EMAPPs come to work (on time), perform a history and physical exam on patients, present that patient to an attending physician, and complete the care. Applicants' skills have already been assessed to some degree by their training programs, but you need to make sure they have the skills to succeed in emergency medicine. When it comes to the position you need to fill, you can be much more specific and objective. Chapter 5 will list a set of skills specific to emergency medicine and EMAPPs. We will use this to create a checklist to rigorously evaluate the skills of each applicant after we've screened out the bad apples. Then, using both analytical and intuitive methods, you will be able to make a much better hiring decision.

For every hour you invest in developing a good hiring process, you will save yourself many hours over in dealing with the consequences of poor hiring decisions. It's time and effort well spent. Your department will be more efficient and more harmonious. Colleagues will be content and grateful for your diligence. Patients will be protected and receive better care. Applicants will not need to go through the pain of pointless relocation or struggle at tasks for which they are not qualified. Hiring the right person means, above all, that you can take a day off knowing that you won't need to worry about what is happening in the ED while you're away.

Hiring and the Fundamental Attribution Error

THE PERSON AND THE SITUATION

What I'm suggesting in this chapter should give you reason to doubt traditional methods of hiring. The idea I'd most like to challenge is that we can use the interview process to find the right person for the job. I'm going to suggest that this is an impossible, unrealistic expectation.

The fundamental attribution error is a cognitive bias describing our tendency to blame behavior or performance on a person's disposition (personality traits) rather than their circumstances. On the highway, for example, we get cut off and make an instant judgment about the driver who did it. And when we are at a restaurant, if our waiter brings us another table's food, we feel we've learned something about that person based on his mistake. Like other heuristic biases, this is the cognitive equivalent of an optical illusion. We look at the picture, and our visual system is fooled because it has evolved to look at real life and real movement, not complex two-dimensional pictures.

Our cognitive circuits are also evolved for real life and for the close social networks where our minds evolved over the last millennium, in tribes. In that environment, it was advantageous to make snap judgments and guess what others might do, all based on what we knew about them. If we couldn't decide what kind of person we were dealing with, predicting what he or she might do would be impossible. Simplifying the process helped us sense danger within our tribe. Making snap decisions helps our brain work faster and with less effort. It increased our ancestors' likelihood of survival in their environment. We no longer live in tribes, but our minds have not yet had time to adapt. Our minds still take shortcuts to help us through already complex decision-making processes that are complicated further by a modern world that is far different from the one our brains adapted to suit. This is for two reasons.

When our minds need to make a complex decision, the tendency is to substitute easier questions for harder ones. We over rely on the guesstimate, which, with added experience, we call the gestalt. Cognitive scientists describe two systems our brains use: the system we use when we need to estimate, and the system we use when we need to make a rigorous calculation. The brain system that effortlessly guestimates is called system one, or the automatic system. The deliberate one is called system two. It's the brain system responsible for long division and other analytical decision making.

Substitution is the bias that happens when we should be using the deliberate system two and instead use the automatic system one. When given a hard question, we substitute an easier one where the answer is easier to estimate. For example, in a dull meeting that seems to never end, someone asks a question that's already been answered. We think, *Wow, that person is not very bright.* It's easier for us to decide that each person's behavior is due to who he or she is rather than the truth: that behavior is extremely complicated and hard to predict and that any number of distractions might cause an intelligent person's attention to wander in a long meeting.

Social psychologists have been looking into this for over sixty years. It's counterintuitive and counterculture in our individualist society. We are not sheep, after all. We want to believe we make our own luck, and in a sense, we do. But the truth is more complicated. And our minds tend to take a shortcut past the complicated parts to simplify reality and make real-time judgements.

PREDICTING BEHAVIOR BASED ON DISPOSITION

Let's get back to traditional job interviews. An applicant sits down, introductions are made, and the interview begins. Some questions are just going over details and logistics, but the interviewer hopes to learn something about the applicant in this conversation. He or she hopes to learn not only about who the applicant is, but also about how the person will operate in the new position.

Will the person be competent? Reliable? Honest? Careful? Manipulative? Dangerous? Will the person steal other people's lunch from the staff fridge?

In 1928, two Yale researchers, Hugh Hartshorne and Mark May, spent five years studying honesty in elementary and secondary-school children. They measured each subject's willingness to lie, cheat, and steal in different situations where they were unlikely to get caught. Would they steal coins from a dish on a table in the classroom? Would they lie to avoid getting a classmate into trouble? Would they lie to their parents? Would they cheat on different types of tests if they thought they were likely to get away with it?

We tend to believe that people who engage in a type of behavior, moral or otherwise, do it habitually. We want to believe that our behavior doesn't vary from day to day. That's why our brains automatically categorize other people based on their behavior rather than their circumstances. Our snap judgements derive from this notion that behavior is consistent. That is why we hope to discover in the job interview how well the person will perform with us long-term. One behavior should predict the other, right?

Hartshorne and May found little correlate (0.21) between dishonest behavior in one situation and that in another. Recall that correlations in social psychology are from 0 to 1, and that 0.6 to 0.9 is considered a high correlation. They reported that the children's tendency to lie, cheat, and steal was highly dependent on the situation rather than a fixed personality trait employed in all situations.

Around the same time, in 1929, Theodore Newcomb evaluated extroversion in boys at a summer camp. He assessed with different measures how extroverted boys acted in different situations. Surely, some assumed, boys with extroverted personalities should show extroverted traits across different situations. Our dispositions all lay somewhere on the spectrum from introverted to extroverted, so our behavior should show some consistency. But Newcomb found it doesn't. Correlations of extroversion across different situations were measured at 0.14. Again, we read this, but we don't really believe it, because it *feels* wrong to us.

Walter Mischel, another American psychologist, later published in his 1968 book *Personality and Assessment*, concerns about the validity of theories about the consistency of human behavior. He wrote that no reasonable (greater than 0.30) correlation had been published concerning measures of behavior or personality testing to predict behavior. His conclusion was that the reason we could not show a link was that there wasn't one. Perhaps predicting behavior was difficult because human behavior was not predictable. It was not consistent across different situations.

What psychologists have been able to measure, and predict, is how misguided we are in our confidence when it comes to predicting behavior. Our confidence is also misplaced when it comes to behavioral consistency. In 1986, Kunda and Nisbett tackled the matter of subjects' confidence in predicting the behavior of others. They recorded subjects' predictions of whether people believed, knowing that a person x is more honest than person y in a given situation, who would be more honest in the next situation. Knowing how behavior varies by situation, we should expect people to doubt consistency. We would also expect them to doubt their ability to predict it, but they didn't. Subjects rated correlation between situations to be high (0.8), when it is actually low (0.2). We over rely on our ability to predict other people's performance, based on what we know about them, because we mistakenly believe that knowing who they are will tell us what they will do. It won't. Knowing who they are, or what they've done, doesn't tell us what they will do or how they will perform more than 20 percent of the time. Overconfidence in predicting performance is based on cognitive bias, and it's an oversimplification. While simplifying helped our ancestors, we need to understand the truth: that behavior is affected by other factors besides personal disposition.

What effect does situation have on behavior? What evidence have we found that behavior varies despite having relatively static personalities and dispositions? Quite a bit, as it turns out. Most people are even familiar with the experimental basis for this knowledge because it formed the foundation for modern psychology.

In 1961, Stanley Milgram tested subjects' willingness to deliver electric shocks to other subjects when told to do so by an instructor wearing a white coat. Regardless of disposition, the subjects shocked people when told to do so, even to the point where the other person seemed to become unresponsive.[1] In 1973, John Darley and Dan Batson sent seminary students across campus to give a speech as part of a similar experiment conducted at Princeton. When subjects were told to hurry to prepare and deliver their speech, the added pressure caused over half of them to ignore a bystander in distress, regardless of the subjects' disposition or religious belief. And in 1971, Phillip Zimbardo had to call a halt to the controversial Stanford Prison Study. This was because some subjects who were randomly assigned to act as guards began to exhibit sadistic behavior toward other subjects who were randomly assigned to act as prisoners. Again, the results occurred regardless of a subject's disposition.

When it comes to predicting behavior based on disposition, psychology says it's complicated and maybe even impossible. Knowing that predicting a person would act in a certain way—honest or outgoing, for example—in one situation fails to predict how they will act in another situation. Recall that there is only a 0.2 correlation of behavior across different situations. It's not surprising that studies of job interviews generally show they predict job performance only about 20 percent of the time.

But the good news is that we are not in the business of predicting behavior. We are trying to find people with skills. Rather than relying on our gestalt during the interview, we should be looking for the wrong people. Those with objectively undesirable qualities can be quickly eliminated from consideration. Then, in the next steps, we can focus not on finding the right person, but on finding the person with the right skill set.

OTHER HEURISTIC BIASES THAT AFFECT HIRING

Confirmation bias and the substitution heuristic affect our ability to find good people in a few other ways.

Our tendency toward confirmation leads us to assume people have had an adequate EM education in their programs or in their previous jobs. We assume

---

1 Recall that in this experiment, the shocks were a sham. No one really shocked anyone. Responses to shocks were simulated using an intercom and actors, but the situational bias had a powerful effect on subject behavior.

they can easily learn the skills and information they've missed while catching up with on-the-job training. This bias is the easiest to overcome. All we need to do is test the applicant. EM core knowledge can be easily and objectively assessed using a short test like the one found in Appendix B, at the end of this book. Feel free to use this short test if you like, but there is also a longer test available online. It's a practice test for the NCCPA Certificate of Added Qualifications (CAQ) that consists of sixty questions, with one that covers only emergency medicine. The cost is fifty dollars.

See: http://www.nccpa.net/PracticeExams?mID=125.

The same goes for the EMR. If we want to know how quickly someone can create a detailed medical record, all we have to do is ask them to do one. Give the applicant a case and watch them type.

EMAPPs also have different levels of customer service skills, which are not assessed in the traditional interview process. Call center customer service representatives are systematically trained and tested, but that is often not the case in the EM world. Assessing that skill set is as easy as any other. Objective test results will tell you which skills you will not need to spend time teaching the applicant. Refusal to participate in testing screens out difficult people who will likely be hard to manage. If you are interested, there are online tests for twenty dollars at https://www.employtest.com (Disclosure: I receive no incentives from the NCCPA or emplytest.com, but I should). OK, so you're not going to have them take an online customer-service test. But I hope you get my point, which is that EM skills, and any other skills necessary for the job, can be objectively tested.

Now, back to heuristics relevant to hiring.

Recall that when we have a hard question to answer, the substitution heuristic is our tendency to substitute an easier one. Math is the easiest example. 46 × 23? It's roughly 50 × 20, which is 1,000, but more precisely it's 1,058. Substitution only gets us close to the truth, and the same goes for estimating competency.

Instead of assuming a provider has a command of wound repair because the person's references did not bring up any shortcomings, test the skill. Have the person sew up a fake wound and quiz him or her on the rationale for the choices made in the closure.

Don't assume that getting through professional school means an applicant has no record of criminal behavior. Pay the money to run background checks, and tell the applicant you will be performing one. Use Google to conduct a search using the applicant's name. A colleague once told me that he was sued by someone they'd hired, only to later find out from a simple Google search that this person had sued all of her former employers (insert expletive). Call all references, and let the applicant know you must reach all of them in order for his or her application to be complete. Don't make any assumptions. And, if possible, directly test the relevant skills using objective methods. This will help you compare each candidate to other applicants. You will be shocked at what you find. And you will be the first to know about the holes in your applicant's knowledge base, instead of the last to know, when these holes create problems.

Some readers might be thinking that they do not want to hire people who just test well. That is a valid point. But you need to know where their skills are at because they will need them to be able to do their job. You owe it to your applicants and the rest of your group to only hire people who have a very high chance of success with your group.

3

How Hiring Emergency Medicine Advanced Practice Providers (EMAPPs) is Different

EMAPPs HAVE VARIED CLINICAL ROLES

Ask directors of twelve different EM groups how they use EMAPPs in their practice, and you'll get twelve different answers. Physician assistants performed 3 percent of US ED visits in 1993, tripling to 9 percent in 2005. The Bureau of Labor estimates the demand for PA jobs will increase 30 percent over the next ten years. NP trends are similar. Some groups use EMAPPs in low-acuity settings, like fast tracks, operating with autonomy. Others have everyone together in the main ED, seeing patients of all acuity levels, with close supervision. Still others have specific rules and guidelines that vary from group to group. Supervision laws also vary from state to state. Be sure you know yours well.

As their roles evolve, there will be growing pains. ED volumes are likely to increase. EMAPP autonomy may not, as increased oversight may be mandated by governing bodies. EMAPPs undergoing a job change may have skills and habits that aren't well matched for their new positions. With roles differing from group to group, much of their experience may be irrelevant. There is also a fair amount of practice variability between EM groups, some based in clinical evidence, and some not. This is another added challenge for EMAPPs starting a new job and for their supervising physicians as well.

SPECIALTY FLEXIBILITY

Unlike physicians, PAs and NPs can change specialty without residency training or board certification testing. The nature of their supervision allows them to flex into other roles. Although flexibility can be positive, allowing for different clinical experiences throughout their career, it also creates instability in the workforce. An EMAPP working in the ED can change to orthopedics, pediatrics, dermatology, or any other field of professional interest to them.

Many PAs and NPs change jobs every three to five years. Half change specialties at least once in their career. The ability to change fields makes EMAPP turnover much higher than ED physicians. The growth in the advanced practice provider (APP) job market means more jobs than trained people will become available over the next decade. Skilled people will be in demand and that will give them autonomy to choose where they work. Training new providers does not make them more likely to stay with your group.

Another major difference between EMAPPs and physicians is the level of training after graduation. Although there are EM residencies for physician assistants, the number of applicants who complete them are small compared to those who directly enter the workforce. The effect of this gap in training, an omission of three to four years of intensive medical training and supervision, cannot be understated. Even the history and physical exam itself, the foundation of any providers' practice, MD or not, benefits from the years of practice and feedback during residency. During residency an ED physician's knowledge base is filled in by thousands of patients and hundreds of atypical presentations. This helps them root out and treat life-threatening conditions in a sea of worried well. Asking the right questions comes from previous missed diagnoses. Unfortunately, this is often learned the hard way.

Residency also offers direct and structured feedback in the form of structured case reviews and morbidity and mortality conferences. These may not be part of most community EM practices. Participating in these programs as a resident helps new physicians learn common patterns of complications in the hospital, and also helps avoid repetition of common medical errors.

THE HARD TRUTH

In the dynamic environment of EM, where time and information are at a premium, new EMAPPs may lack the skill set necessary for independent patient care. The flexibility built in to most APP careers may mean frequent relocation, with job and specialty changes. This makes the knowledge gap more difficult to close. Most training of new EMAPPs is "on the job" and improvised, with little organized structure or evaluation.

EMAPPs

1. change jobs and specialties more than physicians;
2. have a gap in training and experience; and
3. have little organized clinical didactics in most community EDs.

As supervisors, we need to be aware of the gap in training and create situations for our new providers to become well trained enough to succeed. A good supervisor will monitor self-directed learning and require follow-up on cases to foster continual learning in emergency medicine. They will teach skills for real time, evidence-based problem solving, and provide resources to do it, like Up-To-Date and other references.

Of course, if you hire the wrong person, no amount of training or resources can correct your mistake.

4

Finding People Who Are Unlikely to Succeed; Whom to Avoid

PERSONALITY DISORDERS

Borderline, narcissistic, and antisocial personality disorders—all ED doctors know these words. Many people suffering from these tendencies can be high functioning and difficult to detect. One overarching theme among the axis II disorders is lack of empathy, or more specifically, difficulty creating an emotional theory of mind for other people. Recall that the theory of the mind is simply the ability to project another's point of view, and imagine what they may be thinking in a given situation. Emotional theory of the mind is imagining what another person would probably feel in a given situation, a type of empathy.

Lacking this ability can be compensated in other ways, but asking an applicant to self-reflect or self-criticize can help find those who have difficulty doing it. This is one purpose of the traditional interview question: What is your greatest weakness or area for improvement? Everyone has areas of professional difficulty. Asking applicants about theirs gives them a chance to highlight their capacity for self-reflection, a critical skill. If an applicant can't or won't, it's a warning to you that they may lack this skill.

CHRONIC TARDINESS

Although it's unlikely that anyone has ever died from someone coming in late to work, chronic tardiness makes co-workers universally unhappy. There is nothing more frustrating than having a colleague arrive habitually late.

I take that back. The only thing worse is hiring someone who habitually comes in late to work.

This creates such a negative response in the ED that I make a note of telling all my new hires: if you want to be appreciated by your colleagues, come in twenty minutes early, and don't sign patients out for the first year. This advice was given to me when I started, and of all the things we can (and cannot) control, this is an easy one to fix.

The problem comes when we add someone to the team who makes a habit of coming in late on a regular basis. They cite life circumstances and complications, but the truth is that they are showing disrespect to their colleagues. It will reflect poorly on them, and on whoever hired them. Avoid those who can't make it to work, or interviews, on time.

LACK OF ENGAGEMENT/ACCOUNTABILITY

When starting a new job, an employee is the most engaged and accountable they are ever likely to be. Excitement is at an all-time high when everything is new. On the other hand, engagement and accountability are habits. Although some jobs are more fun than others, even wine tasting eventually turns into work. Trust me. Asking references about your applicant's willingness to participate in quality improvement will shed light on the person's level of engagement. Questions about overcoming professional weaknesses will yield information about an applicants accountability.

Many groups don't involve EMAPPs in administrative processes, which is a mistake. When you have nonclinical responsibility, yes, it's extra work, but it also creates a degree of autonomy in your position. EMAPPS can help make their workplace into what they think it should be. It also creates some variation in their work life, adding novel projects. Those who participate in administration, even to a small degree, gain a deeper understanding of the reasons behind policies. It makes those policies easier to tolerate when we know why they exist.

Ironically, rather than making people feel overworked, added administrative responsibility usually helps them stay engaged and stave off burnout. It's all about stoking the hunger for novelty and autonomy. They key to keeping each EMAPPs' administrative involvement positive is to balance autonomy with enough guidance to help make their contribution a quality one.

RECREATIONAL PLAINTIFFS AND CRIMINALS

People who abuse the legal system change jobs more frequently. Therefore, you are more likely to hire them (and other problematic personality types) with greater frequency. They are constantly switching jobs, and are mobile, migratory, and dangerous.

Luckily, legal action, like criminal convictions, can be found, if we take the time to look. A colleague of mine hired a capable physician who later filed a frivolous lawsuit against the group. The suit was so strange that the plaintiff was unlikely to succeed, but it cost the group a lot of time and money for legal fees. My friend's defense lawyer's advice was to settle and avoid further involvement. Of course, that was the new hire's plan from the beginning, but they had not heard any warnings from references or former employees because these people were legally bound to keep silent. In retrospect, a simple Google search on the former employee yielded all the information they would have needed to avoid the pain and expense of the situation.

If you use simple tools to investigate your applicants, you can avoid repeating other peoples' mistakes. A basic internet search and third-party background check will save time and money. It is well worth it.

POOR EMOTIONAL CONTROL

In the emergency department, emotions run high. Emotional control is key to keeping a cool head during crisis. It is also important during customer service rescue, the act of hearing people out after they become frustrated in the ED. Anger, unethical behavior, sexual harassment, manipulation, and the need for an applicant to extensively vent are deal breakers. Congratulations, you've found the wrong people. Now cross them off your list.

The best sources of information for emotional control are people who function under the authority of an applicant. For EMAPPs it's their clerks, techs, and nurses. They can be valuable people to talk to beforehand. Before you contact someone as a reference it's ethically important to get the applicant's permission. But if you can't get permission, because they refuse to give it, that is all the information you will need. It will save you the phone call and you can cross that applicant off the list.

When you do question the references, realize that their response will not be an overt tell-all. Instead, the only clue will be hesitation in their voice. You will need to gently probe deeper with other questions. A hesitation or strange answer is a subtle red flag. Time to cross that applicant off the list and find a better match.

THOSE LIKELY TO MOVE ON AFTER A SHORT TIME

Remaining in the area after initial training is what we want from a new hire. It is incredibly frustrating to go through the arduous process of finding, vetting, and recruiting people who work for two years or less, then quit and leave us with a gap to fill.

People generally relocate to an area for specific reasons. They may have family ties to the area or a spouse's job moves there. Perhaps their recreation has drawn them to the location, or maybe the school quality in an area where they want to raise a family. If the applicant's relocation doesn't seem to make logical sense, it may not.

People try on all sorts of circumstances that are poorly thought out and unlikely to work long term. There is no reason why the applicant's lack of planning should affect your ED staffing. If their relocation doesn't make sense to you, consider taking them off your list. Another applicant who is a better long term fit may emerge if you just spend a few more days searching. If you fill the spot with someone whose chances of staying are fifty-fifty, then you'll most likely be hiring again, soon.

PEOPLE WHO PRACTICE OTHER TYPES OF MEDICINE IN THE EMERGENCY DEPARTMENT

Given the flexibility of the modern APP career, and the ability to switch specialties at any time, you will come into contact with applicants with varied backgrounds. One concern is the applicant who really loves another type of medicine but wants the schedule of the emergency department. Shift work is great and surgical physician assistants can have brutal schedules.

Once hired, these people may have a different idea of how to practice in the ED. Some may want to operate with a greater scope, investing extra time in managing chronic problems, like a primary care physician. This could be beneficial in some departments. Others may not understand that the ED operates as a safety net for vulnerable patients. They may scoff at social work, a vital part of what we do.

Either extreme will disrupt the departmental flow of patients and affect care. It's important to be on the same page about the scope of practice specific to your ED. Often this information can only be obtained from an applicant's former supervisor, so it's important to ask. There should also be data available for the applicant's performance and turnaround times in the ED. Just remember that different departments have different levels of acuity. The numbers should be taken in that context, which you can get from the previous supervising physician.

PEOPLE WHO NEED A LOT OF TRAINING

Finding, vetting, recruiting, and orienting new people is a large amount of work. New grads require structured training as well, but the amount of training differs from person to person. People who easily learn new skills tend to pick up more from their ED rotations than their cohorts, so standardized testing shows where their knowledge base is, and how easy it will be for them to expand it.

People who lack accountability for their learning are unlikely to change when they join the workforce, like those who elect not to crack open the books and begin self-directed learning during clinical rotations. People who have learned how to learn pick things up quicker. They make better use of their resources and can often solve more problems in the ED on their own, rather than dumping them on their supervising physician. In short, they're likely to succeed.

Testing ED core content and asking how applicants like to learn provides a snapshot of where they are and where they're headed. If they seem to be behind, they probably are, and that's unlikely to change. Remember, you want people with a very high chance of success with your group.

PUSHED OUT OF OTHER POSITIONS

Not everyone who has poor job performance is fired. Most have frank meetings with their supervisors, who give them the hint they need to find other work. Applicants with personality problems—those who can't get along with nurses, can't apologize, or can't manage their egos—are often pushed out of their positions. People who are pushed out of other positions are generally risky bets for employment.

> "It was time for me to move on."
> "We had a difference of opinion."
> "It wasn't a good fit."

These are some innocuous-looking phrases, but what they usually mean is, "I was let go for a reason."

Other highly sought-after applicants change jobs for other reasons. They are recruited, they have other reasons to relocate, or they are moving to a nicer area to raise their family. The change has to make sense or there may be something else going on. And in that case, it's time to cross them off the list.

Any applicant who speaks negatively about a former boss is telegraphing a problem he or she had in that position. Those who slam their old supervisors or former work circumstances might change only to find themselves at odds with their new supervisors. Avoid these applicants. The reasons may not be obvious, but there is a cause for every effect.

As stated previously, our minds make us biased when evaluating applicants. We undervalue information we don't have and problems we think are unlikely. We tend to judge competency and fit by how well someone answers informal interview questions. Taking extra steps to introduce objective evaluations will help you find skilled people who are likely to succeed in your group. Listening to your intuition will help you find the "wrong" people, those who aren't likely to succeed. You can then cross them off your list. By using both methods you can make a much better hiring decision.

5

Skills Required for EMAPPs

COMMUNICATOR

While emergency physicians gain permanent autonomy after earning their license, EMAPPs will always require a degree of formal supervision, direct or retrospective. Communication with supervising physicians is a key skill. Patient encounters need to be presented to either the ED attending physician or a consulting physician. This constant need to articulately describe the nuances of each case requires expert communication skills. They need to talk good.

They also need to actively listen and discern. We hear our patients and ask clarifying questions. At times, we teach the patient. But teaching is easier because it is often repetitive and rehearsed. More difficult is the constant synthesis of history and physical data with pertinent positives and negatives, relevant history and working differential diagnosis. Clearly conveying this information is a skill potentially applicable to every patient, which makes it a skill that is highly valuable. People who have it are highly marketable.

In order to clearly organize patient information into a cohesive, actionable presentation from an EMAPP to an attending physician, a few things need to be in place. The EMAPP needs to know, in advance, the differential the attending will consider; then they can provide the right information. If the patient is presenting with symptoms of an acute coronary syndrome, the EMAPP will need to present information relevant to a differential including other life-threatening causes of chest pain, like aortic dissection or pulmonary embolism. They need a command of the EM core curriculum to create a focused presentation. One skill depends on the other.

The EMAPP also needs good organizational skills so that important details aren't dropped. Most high-functioning providers take notes, while others try to hold it all in their memory. Those who write it down recognize that their memory is fallible, and that important details do not always seem important at first. Taking notes empties the working memory and frees the mind to engage in creative problem solving.

Each day, the newly hired EMAPPs will present many of their patients. The quality of these presentations will convey how competent they are to your group. Better presentation skills will smooth working relationships and speed patient care.

COMPUTER LITERACY

With the requirement of electronic medical records comes a new core competency for providers: computer literacy. The faster an EMAPP can learn a new EMR, the faster he or she can concentrate on other aspects of medical practice.

Creating an EMR note for each patient can be labor intensive. Having difficulty typing, navigating the program, or troubleshooting glitches will grind an EMAPP's work to a halt.

The good news is that EMR competency is easily tested. Sit the applicant down to knock out an EMR chart for a fake patient, and it will provide you with a window into the applicant's level of computer literacy, typing speed, understanding of the medical record, and ability to carry out a complex task in a stressful situation.

INTERPERSONAL SKILLS

Patient experience of care is interwoven with medical treatment. When patients come to the ED, they expect not only quality medical care but also an attentive, honest, helpful, and warm relationship with their provider. Failure to meet their nonmedical needs can be disruptive. It will interfere with creating a therapeutic partnership and increase risk of malpractice claims.

EMAPPs should understand this point. They should be able to establish rapport and understand how good communication skills convey medical competency. Applicants need customer service rescue skills for when patients voice frustration. They need to identify patients who need more comprehensive explanations of their care.

When your EMAPP new hire has these skills, he or she can help meet the patient's nonmedical needs without constant assistance during a busy shift. Teaching these skills in real time, on the job, is taxing.

Depending on their level of empathy, some people have difficulty implementing these strategies, even after their supervisors have invested time teaching them. It's better to find an applicant who is already competent in this area.

Another aspect of interpersonal skills is the ability to navigate conflict with colleagues in the ED. Can the applicant resolve a conflict without involving a third party? Is he or she sensitive to the needs of other people on the team, such as nurses, clerks, and techs? Can an applicant convincingly apologize to smooth out rough situations? If not, find someone who can.

PROFESSIONAL DEVELOPMENT

Emergency medicine is complex. Even after decades, it's not uncommon to encounter new problems as an emergency physician. We in the ED need to continue our own education without oversight. Applicants need to be autodidactic.

Finding applicants who can find answers on their own will serve as an investment every time you work together. EMAPPs who start searching for answers on their own come to their attending physicians with more developed questions. Training them in their new position is easier. Spoon-feeding someone who lacks the skills or motivation to find answers to interesting questions takes a great deal of time and energy—time that could be more profitably spent looking for an applicant who already has this skill.

THE WELL-ROUNDED APPLICANT TRAP

Well-rounded applicants are fun to interview. They have interesting life experiences and many talents. They are interesting people, they are interesting to listen to, and so they ace traditional interviews. You need to be able to sit next to them on a bus ride, as the saying goes, to work with them. But you are not hiring someone to ride with you on a bus. If you were, someone small, tidy, polite, and recently showered would fit the bill every time. It takes much more than that when it comes to working together to care for emergency department patients. You are hiring for a specific position to treat patients within your specific scope of practice.

Having a person who is well rounded means they are likely to be somewhat competent in many areas, but the best person will excel in the area specific to your position. Because of this, hiring the well-rounded applicant can be tempting, but it's a trap. What you will find is that these applicants are so interesting many of the staff spend a lot of time talking with them. Then, when it comes to productivity, they may lack the expertise they need to do their job well. They may stay late to complete their charts or struggle to give a clear presentation of a complex patient when the department is already busy. Better to decide exactly what you need them to do and then hire somebody with the skills to do it well.

6

Creating a Position

Carefully deciding the specifics of a position helps avoid the pitfall of the well-rounded applicants, who are interested and excel at many things but lacks expertise in the job you need them to do. Although it might seem that hiring an emergency medicine APP is already pretty specific, your criteria can be further narrowed. The more time you invest in deciding exactly who you need, the more easily you can find a good match.

Doing this will also help you communicate job expectations to the applicants. Some will gravitate toward your position, while others will recognize it as a bad fit for them. Specific job descriptions can also be used to craft performance reviews that help the person you hire know what they need to do to knock their performance review out of the park.

Larger EDs

Most big EDs do more than provide community medicine. They often have training programs, rotating residents, or other administrative duties. Perhaps there is a large fast track that operates somewhat independently, and having an EMAPP serve as its medical director might be more cost effective than using a doctor.

There may be a role for more experienced EMAPPs to teach new hires on a regular basis, or to teach residents in an academic program. Your group may need a scheduler; again, using a physician is more expensive. The good news is that the larger the group, the more flexible the schedule. With more people able to switch shifts, you will have a more stable staffing model. People tend to tolerate being overstaffed better than being understaffed.

Midsized ED Nuances

Midsized EDs have fewer administrative needs than larger facilities. Most have a separate area in the ED for higher-acuity patients, and you may choose to hire EMAPPs with appropriate experience handling sicker patients to staff these areas.

Another important role is orientation of new staff to the ED. Finding the right person to fill this role and also work clinical shifts can help free up your time, if you delegate the task to them.

Quality review is also a good way to teach younger providers, and involving them in the process can lighten the workload. Physicians in charge of chart review can work together with an EMAPP to compile and sort charts, and responses, from providers whose cases are being reviewed.

Needs Specific to Small Community Emergency Departments

Small EDs will have a tighter schedule with less providers working to cover the ED. Their director will need to limit their nonclinical responsibilities. However, they can still do the scheduling, they can be responsible for helping to keep the ED stocked and running, and they can perform other tasks specific to each group.

The important point about customizing a position is to get someone who perfectly fits the role you need them to fill. Extra talents may be expensive and flashy, but overqualified people might just move on.

SPECIFIC COMMON EMAPP ROLES

Worker-Bee EMAPP

When hiring someone to do very focused clinical work, consider the skills required. Productive clinical EMAPPs are self-directed and they need a high level of clinical competence. They do not need expertise in other areas. They do not need experience managing or teaching. They are not being hired to help find and staff the ED. They will need excellent procedural skills and the ability to efficiently communicate with their attending physicians.

Lead EMAPP

Delegating the role of managing the EMAPPs in your group can be a profitable decision. You'll need to find someone with managerial experience, who can skillfully motivate their peers. This will free up the ED director and the assistant director to focus on other tasks. They may be required to attend hospital meetings, interface with other departments, plan for staffing needs, and complete performance reviews. Ours also plans the holiday party. Cheers.

Training EMAPP

EMAPPs involved in training will need to have experience with quality improvement, case reviews, and developing curriculum to teach other newer EMAPPs. They should have teaching experience, and the ability to give negative feedback in a productive way. Another important skill is record keeping, as they will need to keep confidential records for review of cases and performance while remaining in compliance with HIPAA. Ours keeps track to make sure everyone has completed their patient follow-up cards.

As the roles for EMAPPs are developing, it's important to look at your department's needs and realize that, just like MDs, each person plays a slightly different role within the group. Finding the right people for each role increases their chances of success and helps deter people who know they will not be a good fit. Some people tire of low acuity and prefer to work parallel with physician colleagues, whereas others prefer the fast pace and autonomy of working in fast track. Some people have skills that can fill management needs, while others will be better suited to reviewing data.

7

The Score Card

To find the right person for the position you need to fill, you need to know the specific skills, productivity goals, and interpersonal nuances that will work best. Creating a score card helps to collect this information and rank each applicant in an objective way. It's analytical, so it protects you from bias (to some degree). You can move away from the old method of guessing how an applicant will perform based on your gestalt from the interview. Instead, you will create a clear measuring stick to compare applicants, make the most informed decision, and suffer the least turnover.

BEST PRACTICES FOR THE SCORE CARD

Score card items should be actionable. You want to pick skills that can be easily assessed and compared. Putting vague items on the card wastes time. Instead, involve all the people who will work with the EMAPP and get their input. This way you have a group vision of what you need, and you'll know better when you see the right person. This method also engages other members of your group in the process so that when the new members start, they are invested in their success. There will be less hazing. Involve the other MDs, other PAs, RNs, techs, and the secretaries.

The sections of the score card will fall into four categories:

1. Emergency medicine skills
2. Productivity goals

3. Deal breakers
4. Local cultural nuances of your ED

See appendix A for the score card that we use with our hiring, but I recommend you involve your team in making your own.

EMERGENCY MEDICINE SKILLS

Depending on where the EMAPPs are stationed, they will need a working knowledge of EM core curriculum with emphasis on high or low acuity. This can be easily tested with a multiple choice test (appendix B). It's important that the person have an understanding of how to manage the patients' experience of care, as well as how to perform customer-service rescue in the event of an angry patient. An EMAPP's ability to use the EMR, type quickly, and troubleshoot computer problems can all contribute to how likely it is he or she will work out. If the person needs to dictate, that should also be tested to assure competency.

EMAPPs' communication with their attending physician is more difficult to assess. Some applicants have good interview skills but struggle to organize and deliver a coherent presentation. It's difficult to learn. If new graduates lack basic competency, they will need remedial training. To test it, simply give them a patient history, and play the role of the patient or show them a short video. Here is a sample history:

Fifty-year-old male: Yeah, thanks, I came in because I had this feeling in my chest that was bothering me, and I called my daughter about her mother, who is also in the hospital. She said I should get it checked out, so I'm here. It's been there mostly yesterday, and today, sometimes I feel like I might puke, but then it goes away, like when I had my stent, and it's better if I just watch Leno. Last week I was watching Leno, and I passed out, but I didn't get hurt—might be my diabetes. I was out of my pills but refilled them yesterday. What's really bothering me is my legs; they hurt, and I can't go out to get the mail, because it makes my chest hurt.

No, I haven't had a cough or fever, but the doctor asked me that same question last year when I had my stent. I'm not allergic to medicines, but I take Toprol and Metformin. 165/76 108 20 94%RA T36.5

Ask them to read the paragraph, and then present the patient's history to you in an organized way. You should also ask them what they would look for on physical exam and how that would help them form a treatment plan.

Self-teaching is also important in clinical medicine. It will help limit the degree to which your new hire becomes a burden to your partners. Can applicants solve clinical and logistical problems in real time or do they wait for someone to direct them? To test this, give the applicant four clinical problems and ask him or her to find recommendations for treatment. For example:

1. Which antibiotic ear drops can be used in otitis externa if the tympanic membrane is perforated?
2. What is the current antibiotic regimen for community-acquired pneumonia?
3. What drugs can be used to treat soft-tissue infections in pregnancy?
4. What are the five common causes of postoperative fever?

If the person knows the answer, use a different problem. Observe what resources each person uses to get reliable clinical information, as well as how long it takes. If the person starts with Google and ends with an evidence-based answer, more power to them. The person needs to have the skills to solve some important clinical problems alone.

Lastly, as previously discussed, procedural skills specific to your ED are important to test. If there is a problem with the person's competency, you will hear about it eventually, so it's best to find out now. Can the applicant sew up a hole in a pair of blue jeans with surgical instruments? How does it look when finished? And how long does it take? You can cut the leg off a pair of jeans with a hole in it, and have the person pull it over his or her own pant leg. Those who sew it to their interview suit have a problem.

PRODUCTIVITY GOALS

Having a basic idea of how productive the EMAPP should become after six months, and then after a year, will give applicants a concrete idea of your expectations. You should share it with them. Applicants who have poor productivity are likely to self-select off your list when they learn how busy they will be. You can also use the productivity goals for your initial performance reviews, so the applicant will know what to expect. Most groups expect EMAPPs to see two patients per hour in the main ED and three patients per hour in fast track. Ours is more like 1.5 patients/hour and 3.5 patients/hour, respectively.

If you expect them to finish their documentation by the end of the shift, then let them know ahead of time. Some groups expect documentation to be done after the shift and pay people to stay late and finish, while others choose not to do that. You should tell the applicant about your policy. Also, knowing your policy on patient complaints helps the applicants understand what's expected of them.

If the EMAPP will be teaching, you should discuss the number of lectures required, as well as the curriculum load the person is expected to develop.

Above all, make sure he or she understands that you monitor aspects of productivity, and make sure your expectations are understood. Some groups will release an applicant's productivity numbers from a previous job, upon request, in order to help you make a hiring decision. They may also release patient satisfaction data and procedure logs. All of these things can provide helpful information.

DEAL BREAKERS

This refers to specific character traits that serve as the foundation for employment. They are confidential (not shared with the applicant) and might include that the applicant

1. must be honest;
2. must dress professionally;
3. cannot have evidence of a personality disorder;
4. has no history of criminal behavior;

5. shows no evidence of active substance abuse, and
6. must be able to respond positively to constructive feedback.

It is important to know that some state laws prevent you from asking some of these questions, including those about drug and alcohol abuse or medical history. Some of these details are listed in chapter 9, but you should know the laws in your state.

LOCAL CULTURAL NUANCES

Every ED is a little different. How formal are the people working in your ED? When you find someone whose skills fit the job, having the person match the norms and values of your group will make the transition smoother. For example, if your ED has a very social atmosphere, where everyone likes to get together outside of work, will the new applicant feel uncomfortable? Will new applicants get along with your nursing staff? Will the other MDs enjoy working with them?

Geographical ties to an area make turnover less likely. If the person's family lives in Tulsa and the job is in Kauai, how long will that last? People who chronically relocate have long CVs from their constant movement. This is a red flag that you will have to hire again in a few years, after an extensive period of investment of everyone's time, energy, and financial resources from your ED. Again, if an applicant doesn't seem to have a well-thought-out plan for why they are moving to your location, they may not have thought it through. Make sure that it makes sense, or you will be wasting everyone's time.

The score card will need several drafts. It's important to seek input from all members of the team, even if you don't use all of their suggestions. Remember that items should be mostly skill oriented and actionable.

8

Advertising and Initial Screening

CREATING A POOL OF APPLICANTS

If you want a big fish, a large pool of applicants is necessary to find the top-tier EMAPPs. If you find that connecting with the right people happens rarely, then you likely don't have a large enough group of applicants to draw from. You need to cast a wider net. And nets cost money.

Advertising is the most cost-effective way to increase your applicant pool. Groups are often loath to spend money on advertising, and EM advertising is particularly expensive because we are physician groups. But compared to hiring recruiters, or hiring the wrong applicant, advertising is relatively inexpensive.

There may also be free advertising that you can use. Craigslist, PA/NP school job boards, and emailing graduating classes using recent graduates are all free. They're also, quite honestly, low yield. Internet job banks tend to be higher yield because applicants find them easily on Google when they need a job. The three highest ranking on Google today are as follows:

1. Indeed.com
2. Healthecareers.com
3. PAjobsite.com

LinkedIn also has a job board that is somewhat less expensive than other sites, but it still gets a large amount of traffic. Electronic ads tend to generate more leads than print ads. And if an electronic ad doesn't seem to be generating leads, you can usually modify it.

For an ad to be successful, it generally has to be posted for several months—sometimes as many as six months. It is statistically unlikely that you'll encounter a high-quality applicant more frequently than every few months, because skilled EMAPPs don't often find themselves unemployed. They might be looking for your position but don't know it yet, and the timing has to be right, like jumping between orbiting planets. It's much better to wait, suffer a hole in your schedule, and get the right person for the job than rush into a painful relationship with the wrong person. Small applicant pools generally fill from the bottom, with the wrong people first. Only after you have a critical mass of applicants do the best seem to appear.

Using recruiters can be difficult. They are paid when the applicant finds a group and signs the contract. Recruiters get both a finder's fee, and, for per diem, a margin of the hourly rate. This can be very expensive. They may also have lots of applicants for whom they are trying to find jobs. When they sell you an applicant, they are incentivized to find homes for all their job-seeking clients, regardless of skill level. This can be a problem when you are trying to find the best person available.

If you do choose to use a recruiter, then give the recruiter your score card and be very detailed about the position you are looking to fill. Be clear that you don't want to waste time interviewing people who are unlikely to work out. You should also realize that once they have your contact information, they will be cold calling and emailing you all the time. In general, recruiters are low yield and benefit from concrete direction when it comes to filling your position.

TIMING THE SEQUENCE OF EVENTS

Remember, timing is critical when it comes to hiring, which can seem like jumping between orbiting planets. In general, the higher the salary of the open position, the longer the duration of the hiring process for it. Finding a CEO can take two years, ED doctors nine to twelve months, and most EMAPPs four to six months. But once you find a potentially successful applicant, the sequence has to speed up. It is critical that the person feels sought after and not undervalued. The interval between initial contact with an applicant and the screening interview should be no more than forty-eight hours. The initial interview—detailed below—is done over the phone. Then, if things go well, you will ask the applicant for references and set up a more in-depth phone interview, called the CV interview, within a week's time. Assuming that step goes well, references will be contacted and a site visit scheduled, for more focused interviews, within three weeks.

That means that, from our initial contact, we who do the hiring must be prepared to offer our applicants their contract (with their name on it) a month after initial contact. Giving applicants their contract, to look over on arrival, has powerful appeal. Usually, after the site visit, applicants are given two weeks to make their decision. If you don't hear from an applicant for two weeks, it's time to move on.

INITIAL SCREENING INTERVIEW

You place an ad, applicants begin to answer, and you see one that you like and call the person for an initial screening interview. This is the first step to narrowing the large pool of applicants. The call should be made as soon as you know the person is a plausible candidate, no more than forty-eight hours after he or she answers your ad. Prompt contact shows that you're serious about filling your position and serious about that applicant.

Introduce yourself and let the person know you want to talk briefly, for about twenty minutes, and then set up a longer phone interview. Phone screening helps you save time by eliminating people who are unlikely to be top-tier applicants. It's designed to look for red flags, to quickly separate the wheat from the chaff. You might feel loss aversion to screening someone out so soon, but it will save time for you and for them. There will be better applicants.

Tell applicants you have a few questions for them, then they can ask questions, too. Then tell them it should only take twenty minutes, but there will be a longer phone interview later. The truth is that there might not be, and they know that, but this will help them understand that they don't need to tell you everything right now. It's just a screening call.

The questions are simple:

1. What kind of position are you looking for?
2. What do you like to do in the ED?

3. What don't you like to do in the ED?
4. What are your clinical weaknesses?
5. How do you get better at things you don't do well?

That's it. Then open it up for their questions. It's important for the applicant to know that you need real answers to each question, and that you will be asking their former supervising physicians the same questions about them. If they refuse to give you answers, that's a red flag.

Then, after you answer their questions, it's important to find out how much they expect to be paid. This probably seems too early, but it's not. You need to know if they expect a reasonable return for their work. If they don't have reasonable expectations, you're wasting their time, so just politely end it right there.

GOALS FOR THE SCREENING INTERVIEW

The screening interview is a blunt tool designed to screen out the most unlikely candidates. You will have time later to get to know applicants in greater detail and learn about their skill sets. If you move forward to the CV interview with too many applicants, it will eat your time.

Reasonable goals for the screening interview are very focused:

1. Is the person a likely candidate?
2. Are the person's expectations realistic?
3. What is his or her interest level?
4. Are there any obvious deal breakers?

If there are elements of the conversation that raise red-flag issues, save time for both of you and cross them off your list.

NEXT STEPS

After the interview, if things go well, ask applicants to look at their schedule and send you three possible times that would work for them to do a longer phone interview lasting about two hours. (If he or she can't execute this task, then the person is not organized enough to work in your ED). Tell them you will be asking them for more detail about their work history or experience in training, if they are a newly graduated EMAPP.

Also ask for a list of references. Let them know that you will need each reference's personal email address and cell-phone numbers. This will save you time and help the applicant save face. Applicants will feel embarrassed if you can't get a hold of someone because their secretary screens their calls. Selecting the right candidate is an important process, and hiring the wrong person has serious consequences. For that reason, you will need to ask for seven references.

You will need to speak to the following:

1. Any boss applicants have worked for in their work history.
2. At least three supervising emergency medicine doctors, fewer if the applicant is a new graduate.
3. Two nurses who have worked directly with the applicant. If he or she doesn't have their contact information, then encourage phone calls to the former EDs to obtain it. If he or she won't do this, then the person probably won't go the extra mile in the credentialing process or in clinical practice.
4. The remaining people can be character references, but talking to graduating student's clinical advisors is often low yield. They don't always work with the applicant and are heavily invested in selling their student to his or her first employer... you.

9

The CV Interview

After the initial screening interview, you'll have a few likely candidates who go on to do the longer CV interview. As mentioned before, it takes about two hours and allows applicants to tell their story in detail, addressing every line on their CV and more. If the applicant is a new graduate, you will discuss any previous work history and relevant clinical rotations.

ORIENTING THE INTERVIEWEE

Two hours sounds like a long time, but if you're not careful, it can take even longer. The key to getting through all the material is to orient the person you are interviewing. Tell applicants that you want them to tell you the story of their work history beginning with their first job and ending with their current position. Try to account for every piece of time, each year, and look for gaps; explore with polite curiosity.

For each position, ask about the strengths and the weaknesses the person possessed in that position. Ask applicants what their former supervising physicians will say about their strengths and weaknesses when you contact them. Then, when you call these former supervising physicians, it will make the reference-check phone call useful. People who refuse to tell you about their weaknesses need to be encouraged to discuss them. Everyone has real professional weaknesses, and denying them is a red flag. If applicants cannot self-reflect on their weaknesses, then they probably won't seek to improve professionally while in the position you seek to fill.

Next you should ask why applicants left each position for the next one. Here you are trying to find out whether they found a better job or were asked to leave. Some employers will disguise a termination by asking the person to find a new job rather than firing them. Then when you call the former employer they may not be forthcoming with this information. You will need to read between the lines to find out if this has happened to your candidate. It's usually a sign that you should not hire them, though there are exceptions.

DISCUSS THE HISTORY CHRONOLOGICALLY
The applicants should tell their story chronologically so that it's easy for them to get into the flow of storytelling. They will open up more if this happens. Our minds store information chronologically and if you don't allow them to tell the story this way, it will be hard for their storytelling to gain momentum.

Use open-ended questions to get them talking, like "What did you enjoy most about work at XYZ Hospital?" Or "How did you decide you wanted to transition from XYZ Hospital to ZYX Hospital. You'll find, once you do, that people can't help but tell you all the details. They'll talk about friction at work, as well as their struggles. They want to show their best side, but the other stuff is so interesting that it's hard to leave out once you get them going. The details of the story will provide you with concrete data points that you can use in your decision to hire them.

WHAT TO LOOK FOR DURING THE CV INTERVIEW
During the CV interview, you need to learn specific details of the applicants' work history:

1. Was the applicant fired or asked informally to leave from previous jobs?
2. Did the applicant seek to improve professional skills independently?
3. Does the applicant maintain relationships after leaving? Or is his or her past riddled with conflict?

4. When applicants speak about their former positions or clinical rotations, what do they focus on? Are they other-centered? Do they seem dependable and open to the opinions of their supervisors?

Other questions you might ask include the following:

1. Have you ever been formally or informally disciplined?
2. Have you ever had drug or alcohol treatment?
3. Have you ever filed a lawsuit against anyone in the workplace?
4. Has anyone in the workplace filed a suit against you? Were you involved in any legal action? Is there any pending?
5. Have you ever been charged with a crime?

Some questions cross legal and ethical boundaries and should not be asked. These include the following:

1. Are you married?
2. What are your plans for children?
3. What is your religion?
4. What is your sexual orientation?
5. Are you pregnant?
6. Are you disabled?
7. How old are you?
8. Are you in debt?
9. Do you drink or smoke?

Once you finish the interview, you will have a significant history of your applicant that can help you compare him or her to the other fish in the pool. You will also have unearthed red flags on some applicants that can be crossed off the list. You should promptly get back to the applicants who you think have a high chance of success with your group, and bring them out for a site visit.

10

The Site Visit and Focused Interviews

In our group, we have done the focused interviews in two different ways. Both have worked well. Which method you choose will depend on your logistics and your applicant's schedule.

The first method is to do the focused interviews after the CV interview and before their site visit. This way they can relax when they come to see your ED. Also, you can have people who will work directly with the applicant conduct the interview, even if they usually work nights or aren't available during the applicant's visit.

The second method is to do it all at once. This way you can get all the information at once, requiring less time, less focus on logistics, and fewer conversations about the applicant.

The goal of the focused interviews is to engage applicants with people they will work alongside, like an ED tech or nurse, who can flesh out specific issues. They might ask the applicants for an example of how they have used negative feedback to shape their practice style. Perhaps they might ask how they collaborate with their nursing colleagues on medical decision making. Being questioned by a nurse, who you will be working with, certainly sets the tone. This is an excellent way to find people who won't work well with others. They will hate these interviews and probably get flustered. Let it happen now instead of later.

GROUND RULES FOR FOCUSED INTERVIEWS

The most important thing for these interviews is not to repeat the CV interview. You should brief the interviewers so they know the applicant and instruct them not to repeat questions or make up their own. The interview should be only last about twenty minutes, and it should focus on no more than two issues.

Good issues to tackle in these focused interviews include the following:

1. Conflict resolution
2. Customer-service rescue with angry patients
3. Wound care (if interviewed in person)
4. Ability to use EMR (if interviewed in person)
5. Ability to communicate with people below them in the chain of command

Using techs and nurses helps get a different perspective from the people who will really be working alongside the EMAPP. Involving them in the process also helps build team rapport and social capitol.

SITE VISIT

When it's time for the site visit, you want to relax the applicant. This should be a chance for you to show off the good people you work with, rather than your facility. Make sure your applicants are comfortable, fed, and caffeinated. Take them around the ED when it's not too busy and be sure to introduce them to everyone. Most people are anxious about whether they will fit in. This is a chance to show them how warmly they will be welcomed.

Most groups take applicants out to dinner or lunch. It's not necessary to bring the whole group, but you should have them exchange info with a few people so they can ask questions about the group in confidence. Transparency and information help applicants feel less anxious and more at home. Don't keep them out too late.

Recall that, as human beings, we are subject to confirmation bias. It convinces us that the more data supports something, the more likely it is to be true. That is false. One solid piece of contradictory data can prove you wrong. But if you don't look to disprove your idea, that you should hire this applicant or that one, you won't find the reasons, even if they are right in front of you.

This is why you *must* call all the references. You may feel like everything is working out and that the person is probably a great hire. You like him or her and see no red flags. Stop. You must call all the references, and you must ask them hard questions. Without seeking to disprove your intuition, you will only continue to lead yourself down the garden path.

When you call references, refer to the applicants' CV interview and discuss the weaknesses that they talked about when they worked for each reference. Knowing that the applicant brought up their own flaws will loosen the lips of each person and give them permission to be straight with you. For example, *When (the applicant) was working with you, she said that her greatest weakness was _____. Can you tell me about that?*

Some people suggest having references rate applicants on their job skills using a 1–10 scale. That is fine, but you must go further to ask why they gave the person the number. You should also realize that when they give someone a six or seven, it is not a good sign. You should recognize this verbal code of understatement. It's a warning sign.

11

Choosing a Candidate and Closing the Deal

WHICH CANDIDATE IS THE RIGHT CHOICE?

If you began with an adequate applicant pool, the process should now have carved it down to a few solid candidates. Using your score cards and the CV interview means that you now have actionable data to compare the candidates. For your decision, you will also use the opinions of your nurses and techs, who graciously helped with the focus interviews. After all, they will be working directly with the candidate. All this preparation helps provide valuable data that will inform your choice.

Next, sit down with the data and run through it again. Look for any red flags that you may have missed, but also any pieces of data that don't seem to line up. Remember that, in the ED, the skilled become more skilled, and those who lag are left behind. They will be a drain on your busy department. It's always best to pick candidates with the most refined medical and interpersonal skills, but as we will discuss in the next chapter, success has a lot to do with the work environment you create. It's not just about the skills of those you hire. When you get down to a few great candidates, which one you pick matters less. You have already put in the work necessary for success in this part of the process.

CLOSING THE DEAL

Now you have chosen an applicant and made an offer. So much work has already gone into the process that there is a tendency to sit back and wait. The risk is that while you wait for a decision, your lack of contact will be misinterpreted, and you could lose them to another group. What a disaster.

This is the time to concentrate on selling the applicant. You will want to call and check in. Remember the person's spouse may be the one actually making the decision, so you might offer the phone number of another provider's spouse, for a quick conversation. Keep the lines of communication open.

Also realize that candidates *want to be wanted*. Your enthusiasm for having them join the team will positively affect their decision. They will be expanding their decision to other aspects of working with your group. Will they find an affordable home in the area? Will they make friends? How are the schools? Are there activities available that they will enjoy? You should find out what they are concerned about and help them address it.

When it comes to making these decisions, we tend to weigh the pros and cons qualitatively rather than quantitatively. We tend to view additional pros as more valuable, even if they don't add to the overall value. For the interviewer, this can bias us toward hiring a well-rounded applicant who might not be suited for the job. For the applicant, it means that other perks, like a signing bonus, relocation stipend, or concert tickets, will be viewed more positively than a proportional raise in pay. Using a nominal incentive is cost effective and generates lots of appeal.

Whether you decide to offer extra benefits to tip the scale or not, simply continuing to politely contact the candidate will help them understand that you value them. And we all want to feel valued at work.

Long-term motivation comes from autonomy in their work, the chance to master emergency medicine and the chance to make a difference in their new community. Explain to the applicant that, while it's easy to get caught up in the details, your group can offer autonomy, mastery, and work with a purpose.

12

The First Year—Creating an Environment for Success

Staff turnover hurts. It hurts you, and it hurts your group. It creates holes in your group's schedule, adds to the time you need to spend finding candidates, and weighs heavily on your mind when you're not at work. It also hurts new hires who are unsuccessful and then need to find another position. They feel the stress at work when they don't meet expectations. If their skills are mismatched for their position, it can create safety issues for patients. Then, when fired, they need to find a new job and relocate. On top of all this, you will be weighed down with correspondence from their new prospective employers as they call asking for work references. The key to avoiding turnover is to create an environment where expectations are clear and attainable. Then find people who are likely to meet those expectations, and help keep them on track.

BUILDING AN ENVIRONMENT THAT FOSTERS SUCCESS

I assume the reader is also an ED doctor, and I assume we have something in common: in emergency medicine, we are bad at giving feedback to new hires. My first job happened to be a great fit for me. Members of the group and I got along well together and had similar practice patterns. It was busy, but the stress level was reasonable. What I remember, though, was hearing nothing about how I was doing. Was I about to be fired? Did I have any cases where I missed the diagnosis or had patient complaints? Was I succeeding, or was I about to fail? I had no idea.

Having the responsibility to hire and fire the physicians, NPs, and PAs in our group, I have come to a conclusion: I hate firing people. By the time I have gone to the trouble of finding and sorting through them, I grow attached to these people. I'm building a team here, and I like my team. It's mine. So when someone is struggling, it affects me emotionally, and I hate to lose a teammate.

The best approach I have found for preventing turnover and retaining talent is frequent contact combined with clear expectations. Instead of having a hierarchy where information flows only from the top down, we ask the ED staff how our new people are doing. Then we tell them about this feedback. Here is exactly what we do:

Prior to Hire

During the site visit, we discuss our score card with the applicant, and we outline the specific expectations for the position. You can find our score card in appendix A. This allows our potential group member to see what we expect and how they will be measured. If it doesn't line up with their expectations, they tend to self-select and find a position with a better fit. It doesn't feel like this when we lose contact with them; it often feels like we didn't sell them our position very well. But in the long run, it's better to find people with high levels of motivation to meet your group's expectations.

Prior to Credentialing

Next, there is a period of time after the contract is signed and before they start work. Most hospitals have a lengthy credentialing process, and there can be an income gap while new hires are waiting to start after leaving school or their old job. To fill the gap and get the applicants ready to work, we have them work as scribes in the ED, usually for other EMAPPs. We pay new hires half of their salary or hourly rate to scribe, which helps them master the EMR. It also our helps new hires get to know people in the department and become familiar with their colleagues' practice habits. With any luck, the other EMAPPs will give them the lowdown on who orders what and how to approach each attending physician. For us, it's cost effective. For them, it's a head start with no gap in paycheck. Win-win.

I also have each new grad create a didactic program prior to beginning. The one we use currently is EM boot camp, an online course through the Center for Medical Education. *Blueprints in Emergency Medicine* is a good medical student text that we give them, along with the *Tarascon Emergency Medicine Pocketbook*. Get the new hires reading. They're excited to start.

One-Month Review

After thirty days, it's too soon to expect new hires to learn all the details of their new jobs. They are just starting to know the system and probably still getting to know people in the group. Having feedback this early is useful because it sends a message to the new hires that their performance is being judged by everyone. Typically, I send emails soliciting feedback (separately to maintain confidentiality) to clerks, techs, RNs, other EMAPPs, and doctors. Rather than soliciting feedback from everyone in the ED, we focus on the people who work directly with the new hire. I cut and paste the comments into a document without identifiers, then give it to the applicant in a closed meeting. We read it together, and I answer any questions. This helps diffuse interpersonal conflict without allowing it to get out of hand. It also helps generate what is usually a large amount of positive feedback. Your people want you to review their performance. They want to know if things are going well or not.

Open the meeting with positive feedback and let the new hires know you meet with everyone in this way. Ask them how it has been from their perspective: What's been stressful? What's been smooth? There may be more to the issue than what you've heard from others. This will make the review feel more collaborative than one-way, and it helps give you an indication of whether or not the new hire is in tune with the perspectives of the group.

Three-Month Review

One hundred and twenty days is barely long enough to start really getting to know the applicant. The person is settling in and learning the system. But the first year is very stressful, and most of that stress comes in the first three months. When the person knows he or she will get feedback after three months, it makes the stress less unpredictable and easier to handle. The person will do better.

Six-Month Review

After six months, most EMAPPs are hitting their pace (patients per hour) goals and getting the hang of working with their new team. Some get negative feedback. But because this is their third review in six months, it's less stressful, and they handle it with grace. I make a point to tell new hires that the reason for the performance reviews are to help them succeed with the group and help them understand we're invested in their success.

At six months, it's also helpful to begin the process of professional self-development. Ask your new hires what their plan is to continue to learn medicine and improve. Do they have any long-term career plans? What do they enjoy doing in the ED, and what would they enjoy more if they became more skilled? In EM management books, this type of discussion is called professional rounding, and it's usually done on an annual basis. Top providers are driven people. They will appreciate the time you invest in their development.

One-Year Review

After a year, it's usually clear if new hires will succeed or not. If they are unlikely to succeed and you have been reviewing their performance, this won't come as a surprise to them. No one likes to be let go, but you have made it less stressful for them. If they are doing well, then the review is just simple professional rounding.

THE CONCEPT OF FLOW AT WORK

Psychologist Mihaly Csikszentmihalyi has made a career out of studying people's experience of work. He measures the enjoyment of their work during different parts of their routine. Typically, he pages them at different times of the day and asks them to answer questions about how much, or how little, fun they are having at work. He has found that those who are the happiest spend a larger amount of time in a state he calls "flow."

Flow, as defined by Dr. Csikszentmihalyi, is "also known as the zone. [It] is the mental state of operation in which a person performing an activity is fully immersed in a feeling of energized focus, full involvement, and enjoyment in the process of the activity. In essence, flow is characterized by complete absorption in what one does."[2]

It sounds great, and it feels great, but for a task to create flow there are two essential features required. The first requirement is that the task must demand a high level of skill. You just can't enter the flow state playing tic-tac-toe. It's too easy. But knitting, which requires a great deal of skill, won't do it either because it lacks the second necessary element, challenge. Experienced knitters may have challenging patterns, but we need something more. How about competitive knitting for time? Now we are getting somewhere. In contrast to easy tasks that require refined skills, like playing "Heart and Soul" on the piano, flow would require practice and then playing Bach at a packed recital. Tasks that create flow must be skill intensive and challenging. And while it doesn't have *to be fun to be fun*, it can't be easy. Some people call ED physicians adrenaline junkies, but the truth is we are flow junkies.

Csikszentmihalyi believes the key to experiencing flow in the workplace is to develop a worker's skills to the point where the challenging task no longer provokes anxiety. If I tried to play Bach in front of an audience, I think I'd choke. On the other hand, saying the pledge of allegiance would be easy, since I practiced it every day in school. Getting really good at your job makes you less anxious when the going gets tough. Usually, after we start to master a task, we feel a level of arousal because we no longer need to engage in all the cognitive heavy lifting. We only needed that before our skills became hard wired. To get to flow, one needs to go beyond simply competency, to mastery of these difficult tasks. Then you can really enjoy them. Theodore Roosevelt knew this when he said, "Far and away the best prize that life has to offer is the chance to work hard at work worth doing."

---

2 Wikipedia contributors, "Flow (psychology)," *Wikipedia, The Free Encyclopedia*, https://en.wikipedia.org/w/index.php?title=Flow_(psychology) (accessed October 17, 2016).

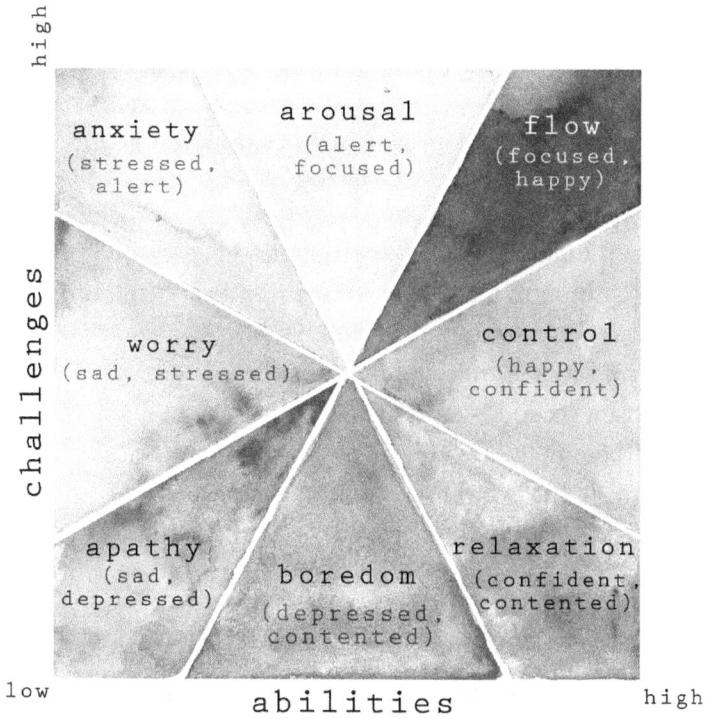

anxiety
(stressed,
alert)

arousal
(alert,
focused)

flow
(focused,
happy)

worry
(sad, stressed)

control
(happy,
confident)

apathy
(sad,
depressed)

boredom
(depressed,
contented)

relaxation
(confident,
contented)

high

challenges

low

abilities

high

Mihály Csíkszentmihályi's model of flow as related to challenge and ability.

During their first few months, I discuss this with our new hires. We want them to love their job and to enjoy autonomy at work. But in order to do so, they need to develop the skills to master the challenging tasks they will perform in the ED. Creating a workplace where they can develop mastery helps us retain talent, and it works better than any other strategy. That, and the hospital coffee, of course.

Delegating and Outsourcing

The method outlined in this text requires a large amount of time. As ED physicians, we don't really have enough time, and the time we do have would be better spent with our families. So how can you make the process more efficient without sacrificing the quality of your new hires?

It's important to understand that there is value in doing the right things and in doing them right. If you need to do it yourself before you can build a team to help you, that's an investment in your practice. Some parts of the process will always be best done by you. For example, the initial phone screening interview is best done by the physician in charge of hiring. You can quickly weed out applicants who are unlikely to succeed. And applicants will feel valued when you call them yourself. Also, before you have adequately trained an EMAPP to help you with the hiring, it's best to do the CV interview yourself. You will want to know exactly what happened at the applicants' previous jobs or clinical rotations, and this will give you that critical information.

Training one of your new hires to help you in hiring can benefit both of you. It helps them have more variety in their work, and some control over who they choose as colleagues. It helps you concentrate on parts of the process without having to do all the work yourself.

Here are some duties that can be easily delegated:

1. Focused interviews.
2. Applicant handling, correspondence, except for the initial screening call.
3. EM testing.
4. Advertising: Spend the money and get a professional to make your ad.
5. ED tours and orientation.

6. Contract questions: Delegate to your attorney; the applicant can contact them directly.
7. Collection of feedback: Keep it confidential, but delegate the process.

Other tasks don't lend themselves well to delegation:

1. Initial contact call—right person at the right time, first impressions matter.
2. Screening interview during first call.
3. CV interview: Can be delegated with proper training but only to someone who will take part in making the decision to hire.
4. Selling the applicant and contact after the process: Final impressions color the entire process, and this is a critical period.
5. Performance reviews.

Using an analytical approach to hiring takes out the guesswork. Involving other members of your team helps create a harmonious workplace. When you invest time in the hiring process, you will save time by avoiding turnover. It also lowers risk to your patients. Outsourcing tasks can also help make the process efficient, but some cannot be delegated. You can build a top-tier team. It will be a great benefit to your group, your hospital, and your community, and your investment in the process will not go unnoticed by any of them.

Appendix A

Sample EMAPP Score Card

Mission: Quickly work with our team to efficiently evaluate and treat patients with a high degree of medical accuracy with emphasis on patient experience of care.

Outcomes:

1. No nursing complaints.
2. No patient complaints.
3. No quality review cases of level 4 or 5.
4. No conflicts with hospitalists or specialists.
5. Two patients per hour productivity @ six months.

Competencies:

Medical:
Scores top quartile of EM test Y/N
Sutures 5 cm wound on pig foot with prep in 10 min Y/N
H&P Presentation skills 1 2 3 4 5 6 7 8
Patient Photos Descriptions accurate 1 2 3 4 5 6 7 8
Learns from mistakes 1 2 3 4 5 6 7 8
Experience with multiple simultaneous critical patients 1 2 3 4 5 6 7 8
Actively participates in CMF 1 2 3 4 5 6 7 8
Tolerance for clinical ambiguity, different ways of treating patient 1 2 3 4 5 6 7 8
Actively troubleshoots system efficiency—i.e., throughput 1 2 3 4 5 6 7 8
Open to clinical feedback 1 2 3 4 5 6 7 8

Professional:
Approachable by RN/Tech 1 2 3 4 5 6 7 8
Professional demeanor 1 2 3 4 5 6 7 8

Skilled communicator with nurses 1 2 3 4 5 6 7 8
Organized communicator with colleagues 1 2 3 4 5 6 7 8
Values/Considers patient experience of care 1 2 3 4 5 6 7 8
Skilled at customer service rescue 1 2 3 4 5 6 7 8
Builds rapport with patient and colleague 1 2 3 4 5 6 7 8
Elevates group morale during times of stress 1 2 3 4 5 6 7 8

Cultural
Articulate 1 2 3 4 5 6 7 8
Honest 1 2 3 4 5 6 7 8
Hardworking 1 2 3 4 5 6 7 8
Friendly 1 2 3 4 5 6 7 8
Helpful 1 2 3 4 5 6 7 8
Curious 1 2 3 4 5 6 7 8
Good sense of humor 1 2 3 4 5 6 7 8
Calm Under duress 1 2 3 4 5 6 7 8
Punctual 1 2 3 4 5 6 7 8

1. Fifty-six-year-old male presents with a sudden onset of sharp chest pain in the right chest with SOB, no nausea, vomiting, or trauma. VS 145/65 98 22 100% T36.2, physical exam is unremarkable. Which of the following will be most helpful in making the diagnosis?
   a. ECG
   b. D-Dimer
   c. Chest x-ray
   d. CT angiogram

2. Seventy-two-year-old female presents with SOB, acute onset, she has lost her medication, and had weight gain, no fever or chest pain. VS 205/76 112 24 89% T36.0. Lungs are wheezy. Which of the following will be most helpful to improve the patient's breathing?
   a. BIPAP
   b. IV furosemide
   c. Nebulized albuterol
   d. Sublingual Nitroglycerin

3. Sixty-seven-year-old male complains of six hours of sudden onset tearing chest pain radiating to his back and a left facial droop. Which of the following is true of the diagnosis?
   a. Aspirin is first-line treatment
   b. Standford Type B is treated nonoperatively
   c. Cardiac catheterization is necessary
   d. SC Lovenox is first-line treatment

4. Thirty-two-year-old female presents with wheezing and shortness of breath. She is out of her albuterol VS 112/67 123 30 88% T37.2 Her lung exam reveals wheezes. What therapies should be considered?
   a. Atrovent

b. Prednisone
c. Magnesium
d. A & B
e. A, B & C
f. B & C

5. Elderly female presents with cough, fever, and chest pain. VS 89/55 121 24 87% T40.1. Lungs reveal rhonchi. Each feature is important when making the decision to admit the patient to the hospital, EXCEPT?
   a. Confusion
   b. Hypoxia
   c. Age
   d. Respiration Rate
   e. BUN

6. Thirty-six-day-old infant presents with wheezing and rapid respiration, siblings have similar illness, but have recovered. Which is true regarding the illness?
   a. The child should be given empiric antibiotics
   b. The child is at risk for apnea
   c. The child will improve with Albuterol
   d. The diagnosis is made by blood test

7. Concerning appendicitis, the value of a normal serum WBC makes appendicitis:
   a. More likely
   b. Less Likely
   c. Neither

8. Forty-five-year-old female with LLQ abdominal pain for three days, no N/V, or fever. Abdominal exam shows mild tenderness in the LLQ without guarding, normal pelvic exam, and negative urinalysis, negative urine pregnancy, WBC is 12. Which is true of the diagnosis?
   a. First-line treatment is surgery.
   b. First-line treatment is Cipro/Flagyl.

    c.   First-line treatment is oral hydration and Flomax, pain meds.

    d.   First-line treatment is ureter stenting.

9. Three-year-old boy presents with sudden onset of peri-umbilical abdominal pain that comes and goes associated with currant jelly stools. Which is true about the therapy?

    a.   Antibiotics are contraindicated because they increase the risk of hemolytic uremic syndrome.

    b.   The treatment is surgical.

    c.   The treatment is air-contrast enema.

    d.   The treatment is oral hydration and antidiarrheal medicine.

10. After a ski accident a young adult male walks home and has a syncopal episode in the shower. In the ED he has abdominal pain in LUQ and a flank contusion. No other trauma is present. VS 75/54 123 16 99% T36.4 What is the next test that should be done after IVs are placed and blood is sent?

    a.   Diagnostic peritoneal lavage

    b.   FAST exam

    c.   CT abdomen/pelvis

    d.   Chest x-rays

11. Which of the following is not part of the evaluation to clear the cervical spine in patients who have had neck trauma?

    a.   Previous cervical spine fracture

    b.   Whether the patient is intoxicated

    c.   Femur Fracture

    d.   Midline point tenderness

12. After a patient suffers head trauma, he is low risk and does not require head CT if he meets certain criteria. Which of the following are one of those criteria:

    a.   No scalp laceration

    b.   Do not take aspirin

    c.   Passed out prior to the head injury

    d.   Did not have a seizure

13. A posterior fat pat typically points toward which type of fracture in children?
    a. Clavicle
    b. Supracondylar
    c. Radial head
    d. Patellar

14. Which feature of low back pain should mandate imaging?
    a. Worse with twisting
    b. Worse with percussion
    c. Straight leg raise test positive
    d. Prolonged use of steroids

15. Fifty-four-year-old male is playing tennis and feels a pop in his right calf. Afterward he can't walk and has swelling of the affected leg. Which of the following is FALSE?
    a. He will need a duplex ultrasound
    b. He should be splinted in equinus
    c. He should be made nonweight bearing
    d. He is unlikely to get compartment syndrome

16. What is the current recommendation for two-year-olds with uncomplicated acute otitis media?
    a. Oral Amoxicillin, unless penicillin allergic
    b. Topical antibiotic ear drops
    c. Forty-eight-hour home surveillance, with no treatment
    d. Oral cephalosporin, unless allergic

17. Patients with epistaxis and bilateral anterior-posterior balloons should:
    a. Have next-day ENT follow up
    b. Have their coagulation studies PT/PTT tested in the ED
    c. Be admitted on a cardiac monitor

18. Twenty-three-year-old male with a dental abscess had a firm woody mass under his tongue. What is the optimal treatment?

a. Oral antibiotics
b. Referral to ENT and oral antibiotics
c. IV antibiotics and referral to ENT
d. Admission and possible intubation, with IV antibiotics
e. None of the above

19. Eighteen-year-old female left her contact lenses in overnight and now presents with blurred vision and unilateral eye pain. Vision is 20/20 right eye and 20/80 left eye. Slit lamp shows a white 2 mm lesion at six o'clock position on the cornea with fluorescein uptake. Which therapy is recommended?
a. Lacrilube twice daily
b. Bacitracin eye ointment twice daily
c. Ciloxan q two hours while awake
d. Vigamox four times a day
e. None of the above

20. Thirty-four-year-old female presents with acute headache, vomiting, and photophobia after a movie; what test is indicated?
a. Head CT
b. Lumbar puncture
c. ESR
d. Tonometry
e. None of the above

21. Five-year-old male is brought in by his parents who are concerned he took an unknown amount of Tylenol. What is the best plan?
a. Admission for liver-function-test monitoring
b. Serial Tylenol levels every two hours ×3
c. Treatment with oral N-acetylcysteine and admission
d. Four-hour post ingestion Tylenol level

22. Twenty-one-year-old female is brought in by friends after she gets drunk on her birthday. Which of the following will speed her clearance of alcohol?

a. IV Normal Saline
b. Banana bag
c. Caffeine
d. Eating a high-carbohydrate meal
e. None of the above

23. Which drug is the antidote to a heroin overdose?
   a. Flumazenil
   b. Naloxone
   c. N-Acetylcysteine
   d. Amyl Nitrite
   e. None of the above

24. Which of the following can be used to irrigate a wound?
   a. Tap water
   b. Betadine
   c. Chlorhexidine
   d. Hydrogen Peroxide
   e. None of the above

25. Lacerations in which location should not be anesthetized using lidocaine with epinephrine?
   a. Scalp
   b. Thigh
   c. Wrist
   d. Heel
   e. Nose

26. Which suture is best for facial wounds?
   a. 3-0 Silk
   b. 6-0 Nylon
   c. 4-0 Proline
   d. 4-0 Cat Gut
   e. 5-0 Silk

27. Patients with meningitis may have:
    a. Neck stiffness
    b. Fever
    c. Seizure
    d. Altered mental status
    e. Any of the above

28. Which of the following is an alternative treatment to MRSA in patients allergic to sulfa drugs?
    a. Bactrim
    b. Keflex
    c. Doxycycline
    d. Augmentin
    e. Cipro

29. Which, other than steroids, is the treatment for severe croup?
    a. Albuterol
    b. Racemic Epinephrine
    c. Amoxicillin
    d. Amantidine
    e. None of the above

30. Patients with suspected pertussis should:
    a. Be admitted to the hospital
    b. Be treated empirically with azithromycin
    c. Be treated empirically with amoxicillin
    d. Be vaccinated within seventy-two hours

31. Three-year-old female presents to the ED with vomiting and diarrhea. She is found to have a blood sugar of 36. Why is this?
    a. The patient was given insulin by someone and needs admission for child abuse.
    b. The patient is diabetic.
    c. The patient likely ingested an oral hypoglycemic.

d. The patient has ketotic hypoglycemia.
e. None of the above.

32. Twenty-four-year-old female with cervical motion tenderness caused by an infection requires:
a. Cipro
b. Vantin
c. Azithromycin
d. Rocephin
e. Flagyl

33. Nineteen-year-old female presents with vaginal bleeding, abdominal cramping, and syncope. On exam her cervical os is closed, and her abdomen is soft and mildly tender. She has a beta-HCG of 1645 and an ultrasound that shows no adnexal mass, no free fluid, and no IUP. What is the best course of action?
a. Admission for laparotomy
b. CT scan
c. Forty-eight-hour OBGYN follow up for repeat beta-HCG
d. Repeat ultrasound in forty-eight hours

34. Four-year-old boy presents with unilateral testicular pain? What is the best initial test?
a. Urinalysis
b. Renal ultrasound
c. Testicular ultrasound
d. CT KUB without contrast

35. Asymmetric pupils in the absence of trauma are concern for all of the following EXCEPT:
a. Increased intracranial pressure and herniation
b. Multiple sclerosis
c. Posterior communicating artery aneurysm
d. Afferent pupillary defect

36. Hypotension, jugular venous distension, and muffled heart sounds indicate:
    a. Cardiac Contusion
    b. Pulmonary Contusion
    c. Pericarditis
    d. Cardiac Tamponade

37. Treatment of carbon-monoxide poisoning includes:
    a. IV fluids
    b. Screening for cardiac ischemia
    c. Oxygen
    d. Bronchoscopy

38. A two-year-old has swallowed a button battery. On radiograph it is in the stomach. Which is the treatment of choice?
    a. Emergency endoscopy
    b. Surgical consultation
    c. Oral charcoal with sorbitol
    d. Twenty-four-hour follow up for repeat x-ray

39. Pregnant patients need Rhogam administration if they:
    a. Are Rh+ and have vaginal bleeding
    b. Are Rh− and have vaginal bleeding
    c. Are Rh+ but have no vaginal bleeding
    d. Are Rh− but have no vaginal bleeding

40. Twenty-four-year-old male has fever and a rash five weeks after resolution of a painless penile ulcer. What is the treatment of choice?
    a. Acyclovir
    b. Penicillin
    c. Azithromycin
    d. IM Rocephin

41. After a head injury, a patient has bilateral black eyes. This raises concern for:
    a. Basilar skull fracture

b. Subdural hematoma
c. Epidural hematoma
d. Temporal skull fracture

42. Calcaneus fractures are at risk for:
   a. Compartment syndrome
   b. Lumbar fracture
   c. Malunion
   d. All of the above

43. A patient suffering from heroin addiction and skin infection is at risk for:
   a. Septic joint
   b. Endocarditis
   c. Nephritis
   d. Rhabdomyolysis

44. Zone 2 neck injuries deep to the platysmus require:
   a. Surgical exploration
   b. Wound care and closure
   c. Healing by secondary intention
   d. Plastic surgery consultation

45. Ebola is transmitted:
   a. Airborne
   b. Oral Secretions
   c. Blood borne
   d. All of the above

46. A bradycardic patient who consumed a garden herb is best stabilized with which medication?
   a. Epinephrine
   b. Dopamine
   c. Norepinephrine
   d. Atropine

47. A patient with substernal dull chest pain made worse by lying flat with malaise is most descriptive of which condition?
   a. Pulmonary embolism
   b. Congestive heart failure
   c. Pneumonia
   d. Pneumothorax
   e. Pericarditis

48. An elderly woman is tender at the pubic symphysis after a fall. She most likely suffered a(n):
   a. Femoral neck fracture
   b. Intertrochanteric hip fracture
   c. Inferior rami fracture
   d. Acetabular fracture

49. Free air in the abdomen can indicate all of the following except:
   a. Recent laparoscopy
   b. Peptic ulcer
   c. Diverticulitis
   d. Appendicitis

50. The diagnosis of compartment syndrome is made with:
   a. CT scan
   b. Striker needle insertion
   c. MRI
   d. Ankle brachial index

EM Core-Content Answers

1. C	18. D	35. A
2. A	19. C	36. D
3. B	20. D	37. C
4. E	21. D	38. A
5. B	22. E	39. B
6. B	23. B	40. B
7. C	24. A	41. A
8. B	25. E	42. D
9. C	26. B	43. B
10. B	27. E	44. A
11. A	28. C	45. C
12. D	29. B	46. D
13. B	30. B	47. E
14. D	31. D	48. C
15. A	32. D	49. D
16. C	33. A	50. B
17. C	34. C	

Appendix C

Urgent Care Test

1. Sixty-year-old female presents with chest pain that is sharp, worse with deep breath, and associated with hemoptysis. Which is the most likely diagnosis?
   a. ACS
   b. Aortic dissection
   c. Pneumonia
   d. Pulmonary embolism
   e. Pneumothorax

2. Twenty-year-old female has syncope. All of the following may be the cause EXCEPT:
   a. Pulmonary embolism
   b. Ectopic pregnancy
   c. Subarachnoid hemorrhage
   d. Pneumothorax
   e. GI Bleed

3. Which of the following rhythms must be immediately treated by a cardiologist?
   a. Bigeminy
   b. First-degree atrioventricular block
   c. Complete heart block
   d. Sinus arrhythmia
   e. Sinus pause

4. Respiratory Syncytial Virus associated wheezing typically responds to albuterol nebulizing treatments.
   a. True
   b. False

5. Six-month-old male with purulent-green nasal discharge may be suffering from sinusitis.
   a. True
   b. False

6. Otitis media can be treated with home observation and no antibiotics in some cases.
   a. True
   b. False

7. Six-month-old male falls out of a shopping cart and hits his head, then vomits twice after crying. Which is true?
   a. The child may be discharged with next day primary care follow-up.
   b. Head CT is indicated.
   c. MRI is indicated.
   d. Admission to pediatrics for observation is indicated.
   e. None of the above.

8. Four-year-old with a volar displaced radius and ulnar fracture presents. This fracture is called:
   a. Colle's fracture
   b. Smith's fracture
   c. Bennet's fracture

9. Finger dislocations require:
   a. Surgery to repair the volar plate
   b. Surgery to explore for tendon injury
   c. Volar splinting
   d. Dorsal splinting

10. Which of the following is not a sign of infectious tenosynovitis?
    a. Joint irritability

    b. Pain over tendon sheath

    c. Pain with passive extension

    d. Sausage digit

11. What is the treatment for mallet finger?

    a. Surgical consultation

    b. Reduction

    c. Splinting

12. What is the treatment of a Dancer's fracture?

    a. Casting

    b. Boot orthotic

    c. Postop shoe

    d. Surgery

13. Chance fractures involve:

    a. The metatarsals

    b. The calcaneus

    c. The talus

    d. The lumbar vertebrae

    e. The tibia

14. Calcaneal fractures are splinted with:

    a. Bulky Jones splint

    b. Stir-up splint

    c. Short-leg posterior splint

    d. Boot orthotic

    e. Postop shoe

15. Corneal infections from contact lens scratch are at risk for:

    a. *E. coli*

    b. MRSA

   c. Pseudomonas
   d. Streptococcus
   e. Yersinia

16. *E. coli* enteritis puts children at risk for:
   a. Mesenteric adenitis
   b. Hemolysis
   c. Septic arthritis
   d. Peptic ulcers

17. Symptoms of nephritis in children include all of the following EXCEPT:
   a. Dysuria
   b. Urine casts
   c. Facial swelling
   d. Scrotal swelling
   e. Dark cola-colored urine

18. Infected uretolithiasis requires:
   a. IV antibiotics
   b. Stenting + IV antibiotics
   c. Lithotripsy + IV antibiotics
   d. Surgery + IV antibiotics
   e. Cystoscopy + IV antibiotics

19. Elderly patient develops frothy yellow diarrhea after being treated for a sinus infection with Augmentin. Which is the treatment of choice?
   a. IV fluids
   b. Lomotil
   c. Vancomycin
   d. Clindamycin

20. What is the treatment for pelvic inflammatory disease?
   a. Rocephin 125 mg IM, Azithromycin 1 gram PO

    b.   Rocephin 250 mg IM, Azithromycin 1 gram PO

    c.   Rocephin 1 gram IV, Azithromycin 1 gram PO

    d.   Rocephin 250 mg IM, Doxy 100 mg BID × 10 days PO

    e.   Rocephin 250mg IM, Vantin 300 mg PO

21. Which STD can cause polyarticular arthritis when left untreated?
    a. Chlamydia
    b. Syphilis
    c. Hemophylis ducreyi
    d. Herpes simplex 2
    e. Gonorrhea

22. Which STD typically causes abdominal pain in the early stages of infection?
    a. Bacterial vaginosis
    b. Herpes simplex 2
    c. Chlamydia
    d. Trichomonas

23. If a patient is diagnosed with a sexually transmitted infection, you may write him a prescription for his sexual partner without his partner signing in for treatment.
    a. True
    b. False

24. Which disease is characterized by vertigo after viral infection?
    a. Meniere's disease
    b. Benign paroxysmal positional vertigo
    c. Vertebrobasilar insufficiency
    d. Labyrinthitis
    e. Acoustic neuroma

25. The rash associated with which disease blanches with palpation?
    a. Meningitis

b. Parvovirus B19

c. Vasculitis

d. Henoch Schonlein Purpura

e. Thrombocytopenia

26. What is the standard of care for abscess treatment?
    a. Oral Bactrim and warm compress
    b. Incision and drainage without antibiotics
    c. Incision and drainage with oral Bactrim

27. Sixteen-year-old female presents with syncope and diaphoresis. VS 76/34 146 26 36.9 100%RA. Her BP after 1 liter is lower at 65/32. Hemoglobin is 13. Which treatment is best?
    a. IV antibiotics
    b. Blood transfusion
    c. IM epinephrine
    d. IM Benadryl
    e. IV Norepinephrine

28. Urticaria can be caused by all of the following EXCEPT:
    a. Cold weather
    b. Autoimmune disease
    c. New detergent
    d. Tinea corporis
    e. Shellfish

29. Two-year-old male presents with a limp. Which of the following is least likely?
    a. Ankle sprain
    b. Slipped capital femoral epiphysis
    c. Septic hip
    d. Tibial spiral fracture

30. What suture is typically used for intraoral lacerations?
    a. Nylon

b. Vicryl
c. Chromic gut
d. Silk

31. Which of the following medicines for UTI can cause renal failure?
   a. Cipro
   b. Macrodantin
   c. Keflex
   d. Bactrim
   e. Amoxicillin

32. What is the drug of choice for hyperkalemia with QRS widening?
   a. Kayexylate
   b. Sodium Bicarbonate
   c. Lasix
   d. Albuterol
   e. Glucagon

33. Which medicine does not potentiate Coumadin dosing?
   a. Cipro
   b. Rifampin
   c. Cimetidine
   d. Macrodantin

34. Thirty-four-year-old male is suffering from GERD. Ranitidine has not re-solved his symptoms. What can be recommended?
   a. Addition of omeprazole
   b. Replacement of ranitidine with omeprazole
   c. Addition of sucralfate
   d. Addition of Maalox

35. Which drug for MRSA can be given to pregnant patients?
   a. Bactrim
   b. Clindamycin

c. Vancomycin
d. Keflex
e. Doxycycline

36. Concerning rashes, a target lesion suggests:
    a. MRSA
    b. Lyme disease
    c. Varicella
    d. Tinea corporis
    e. Contact dermatitis

37. Patients with traumatic hyphema are at risk for:
    a. Increased intraocular pressure
    b. Infection
    c. Corneal ulcer
    d. Globe rupture

38. Second-degree acromioclavicular separation requires:
    a. Orthopedic surgery
    b. Reduction
    c. CT scan of the shoulder
    d. Pain control and sling

39. Sudden onset of sharp chest pain, dyspnea, and fever is classic for:
    a. Acute myocardial infarction
    b. Pulmonary embolism
    c. Pneumonia
    d. Empyema

40. Facial weakness from Bell's palsy spares the forehead.
    a. True
    b. False

41. Painless jaundice is concerning due to:
    a. Hepatitis
    b. Ascending cholangitis
    c. Choledocholithiasis
    d. Pancreatic neoplasm
    e. Pancreatitis

42. Acute glaucoma is treated with:
    a. Lateral canthotomy
    b. Pilocarpine
    c. Lasix
    d. Trabeculectomy
    e. Marijuana

43. Female pelvic pain that is positional, sudden onset, and associated with vomiting is classic for:
    a. Torsion
    b. Ectopic
    c. Kidney stone
    d. Appendicitis

44. Diabetic Ketoacidosis is characterized by all of the following EXCEPT:
    a. Pseudohyponatremia
    b. Global hypokalemia
    c. Hyperglycemia
    d. Hypercalcemia

45. Digital blocks require epinephrine to be effective.
    a. True
    b. False

46. Priapism is treated with all of the following except:
    a. Terbutaline

b. Needle drainage
c. Phenylephrine
d. Benadryl

47. Tearing chest pain that radiates to the scapula is classic for:
    a. Aortic dissection
    b. Biliary colic
    c. Myocardial infarction
    d. Pneumothorax

48. Sciatica in patients with prostate cancer requires:
    a. Steroids
    b. Pain medications
    c. Emergency MRI
    d. Oncology follow-up

49. The second most common carpal bone fracture is the:
    a. Scaphoid
    b. Trapezium
    c. Capitate
    d. Triquetrum

50. Compartment syndrome is treated with:
    a. Needle aspiration
    b. Fasciotomy
    c. Elevation
    d. Ice

Urgent Care Test Answers

1. D	24. D	47. A
2. D	25. B	48. C
3. C	26. B	49. D
4. B	27. C	50. B
5. B	28. D	
6. A	29. A	
7. B	30. C	
8. B	31. D	
9. C	32. B	
10. A	33. D	
11. C	34. B	
12. C	35. B	
13. D	36. B	
14. A	37. A	
15. C	38. D	
16. B	39. B	
17. A	40. B	
18. B	41. D	
19. C	42. B	
20. D	43. A	
21. E	44. D	
22. A	45. B	
23. A	46. D	

Acknowledgments

First, I would like to thank my gracious wife for allowing me the time to finish this work. She is patient, kind, and brilliant. Also, I feel that Vivian Chen did an excellent job on the cover and illustrations. Thanks to the PAs in our group for crash testing the tests for me, just plain old-fashioned fun. Lee Ross and Richard Nesbitt wrote a book called *The Person and the Situation* that has changed the way I look at the world and the way I hire people. I feel immense gratitude for their dedication to the field of psychology and for their willingness to put their findings in print in a format I can understand as a layperson. Thanks to my boys—I'll come and play as soon as this is done. Thanks to my colleague and mentor Harry Kleiner, who has helped me become a better doctor, father, and colleague.

About the Author

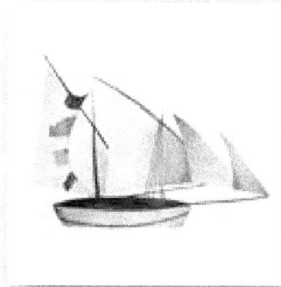

Gary Josephsen is a community emergency physician practicing full-time clinical medicine. He also serves as an affiliate professor with Oregon Health Sciences University, teaching physician assistant students in his community ED. He lives in Oregon with his wife and two boys. They spend their days playing in the woods while it rains.

www.ingramcontent.com/pod-product-compliance
Lightning Source LLC
Chambersburg PA
CBHW061300220326
41599CB00028B/5719